LIVE THROUGH THIS

Cheryl and Janet Snell

© 2017 Scattered Light Library
ISBN 10: 149617559X
ISBN 13: 9781496175595
Live Through This
Cheryl Snell
Janet Snell

Acknowledgments

Thanks to the editors of the journals in which these poems first appeared, sometimes in altered forms: *Catastrophe's Cusp* in Wicked Alice, *Grief* in Ithaca Lit, *Support Group* in PANK, *Where We Started From* and *Operating Theater* in Red Booth Review, *Circle Theory* in Boston Literary Review, *Know, Recovery Room, Faith, Late Effects* in Verse Wrights, *Aggressive* in The Curator, *No Second Acts* in Olentangy Review, *Radiation* in Egg, *Recurrence* in Deep Water Literary Journal, *Anniversary of Our Escape* in Red River Review, and *Afterimage* in The Inflectionist Review.

Poems

Live Through This

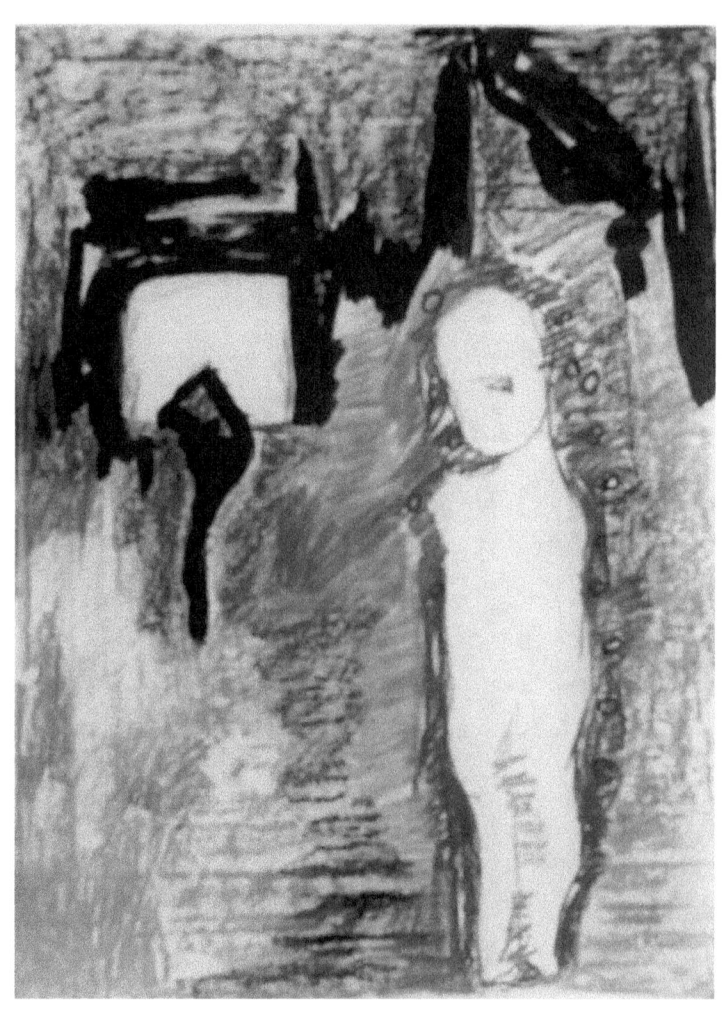

Catastrophe's Cusp

The day you trip down the stairs
spill coffee on shower-scalded skin
crash the car on the way to the ER
and return to a kitchen where
the bleeding never stops, there is
a burglar with an itchy trigger finger
lurking on the Welcome mat.

He watches you misdial 911
and when a voice impersonating the bank
comes on to steal your identity
before some pack of marauding cells can
explain that you're invisible already
a shadow mortared to the wall
of an unfurnished room.

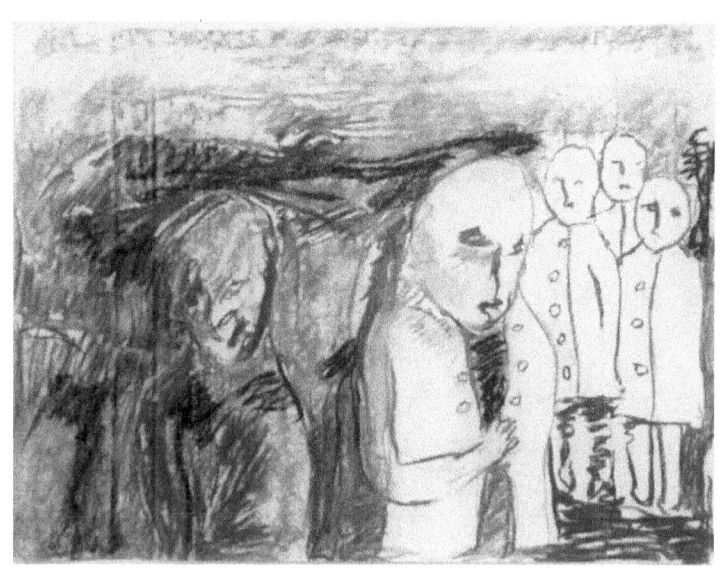

Know

We won't know
  until the biopsy
      the labs come back
        we get in there.

As if danger can only be known
by its face, not shape
    not shadow.

What we do know
is that much worse will come—
the mass unzipped and appraised
the scar's mad map burning skin inward.
And when you unbutton your blouse
for yet another white-coated crowd
you'll surrender
like the nude at Manet's picnic
no longer listening to talk
of cure and recurrence
risk and benefit,
prediction and the probability
that all this is necessary
because *we just never know.*

9

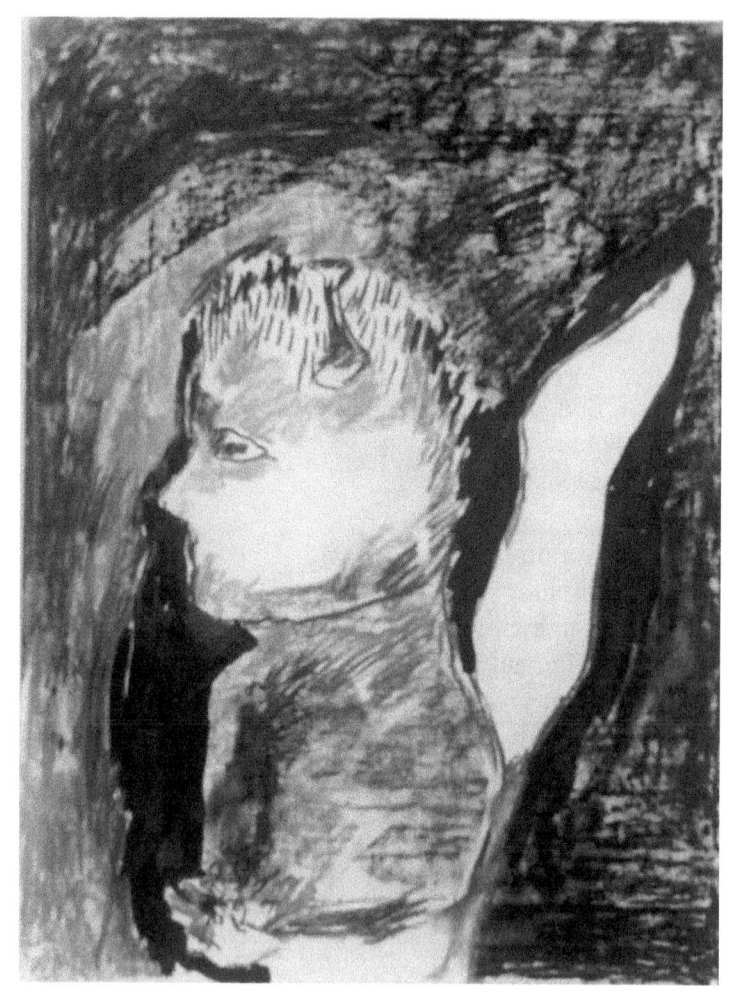

Grief

It's in the details:
you standing
on the other side
of your snapped connection
waiting for the static
to subside. It's not as if
the pain could burn you
tattoo lightning across your back
although that's what
it feels like at first. Instead
the sensation leafs out
flares in the mind
with echoes bridging
one thought to another
like those beaded necklaces
you made as a child
their painted gleam
flaking off in your palm
long before the future arrived
to slip right through your fingers..

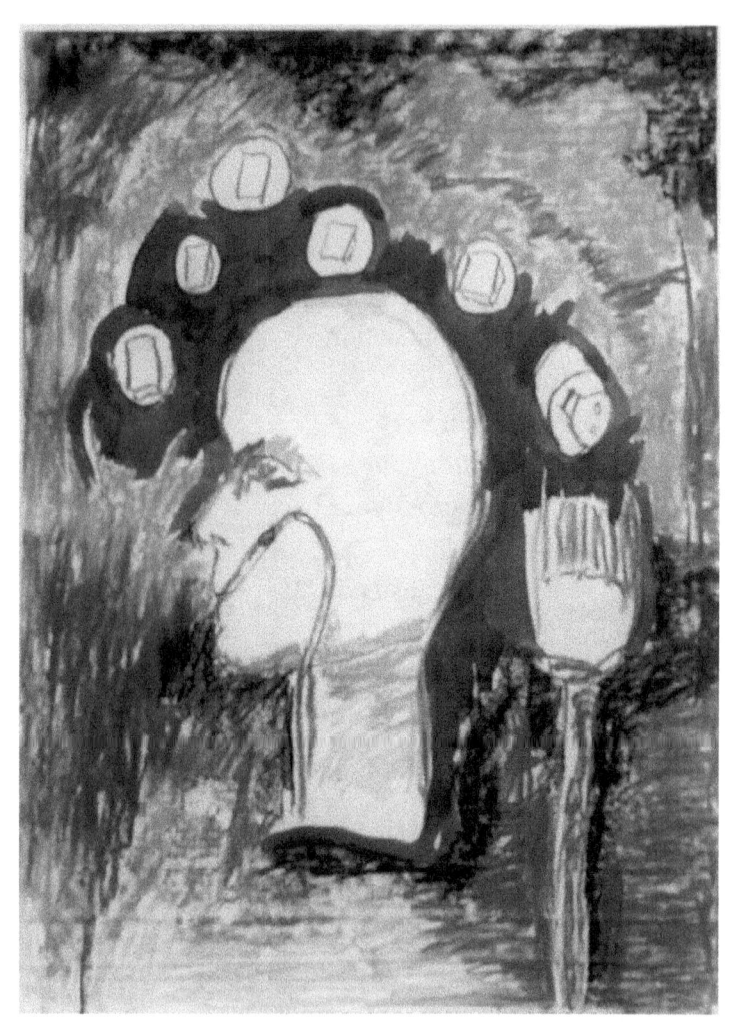

Bad Fit

what doesn't fit
sticks like a key
in a rusted lock
breaking off
fact from theory
impulse from forethought
bad days from worse nights
the space between
ambulance and overpass
a square peg in a round hole
a big pill down a narrow throat
a paper gown over gooseflesh
a plastic ID on a thin wrist
holding in the urge to flee

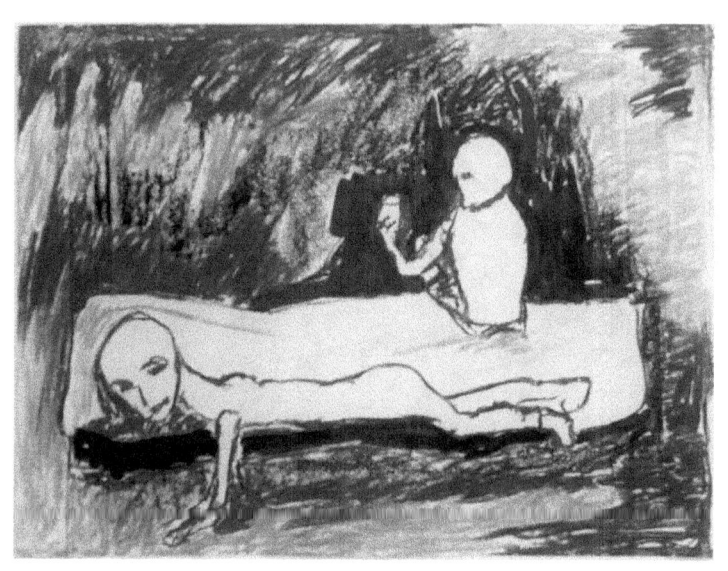

Neither Nor

The hospital
its electric fires
and crossed wires
is not mere metaphor
for a patient's glitches.
Nor its complex grids
its pill bottle lids
the disconnect of its
off/on switches.

Before the cancer
you never intend
to surrender.
Nor is it unheard of
to crawl
on your belly
toward bed's edge
after.

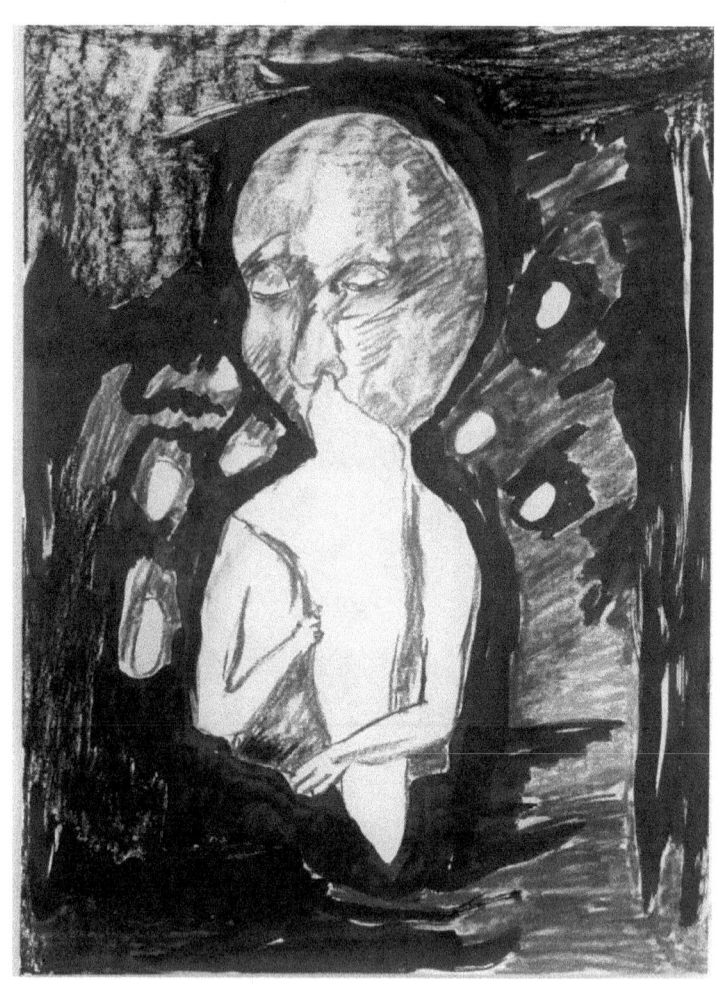

Advance Directive

You bargain for time
until it lets you close your eyes.

Some want to be remembered only
until their scent fades from the sheets

or the disc of camphor crumbles unlit
in the lamp; others want to last

until their gestures freeze and turn tacit
loosing them into the landscape where

stars were last seen, each one blowing
its fuse, the plunging light erasing the sky.

Sign this, and someone else will decide
when your planets unravel like string

a knot of scars on the verge of change
unpredictable as a wayward cell.

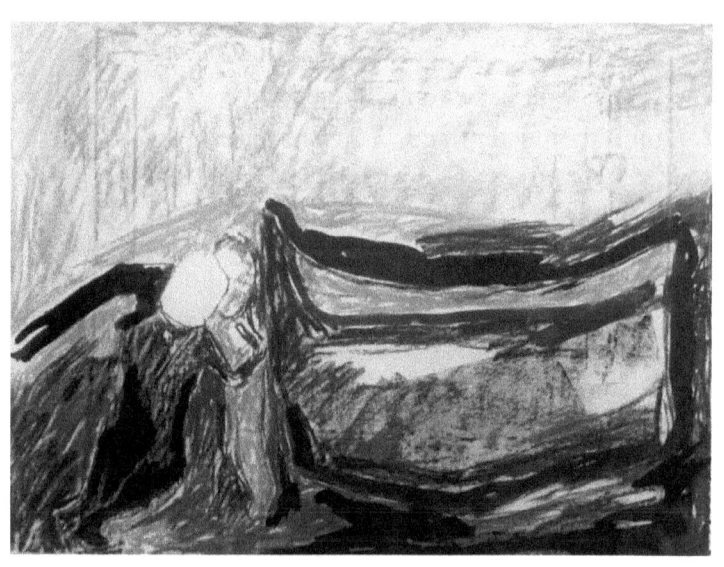

Anesthesia

The dream a dive
to the bow
of a sinking ship

Fearless deft diver
scalpel gleaming
in his teeth

Fearless deft scalpel
freeing the carved woman
from a ship already drowned

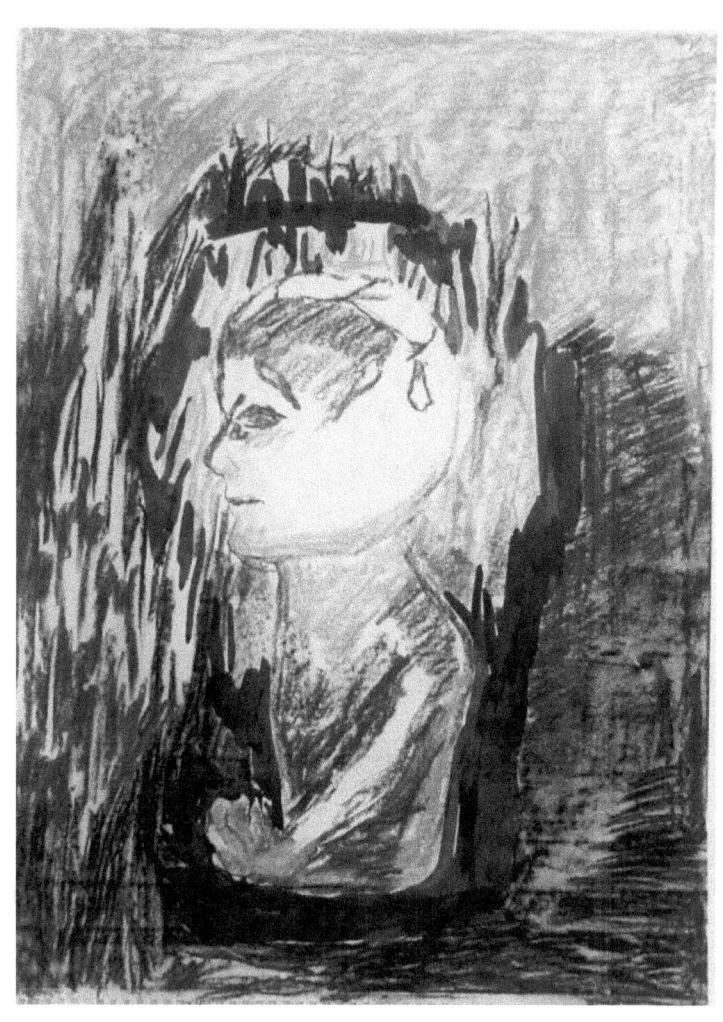

Operating Theater

This is the moment
you are most alone
systems thudding, breath
stretching to nothing.
A moment before
a tear made of the day
escaped like the slow start of rain
and your fingers curled slightly.
Around what? Machine sounds
doppler away, also refusing to be held.
There's no fear of the numbness
that creeps through you now.
Let it come
loosening muscle, thinning thought.
At this moment, the mind talks in riddles
its language a mystery that leaves you
breathless and broken over the oblivion
that has traveled so far to touch you.

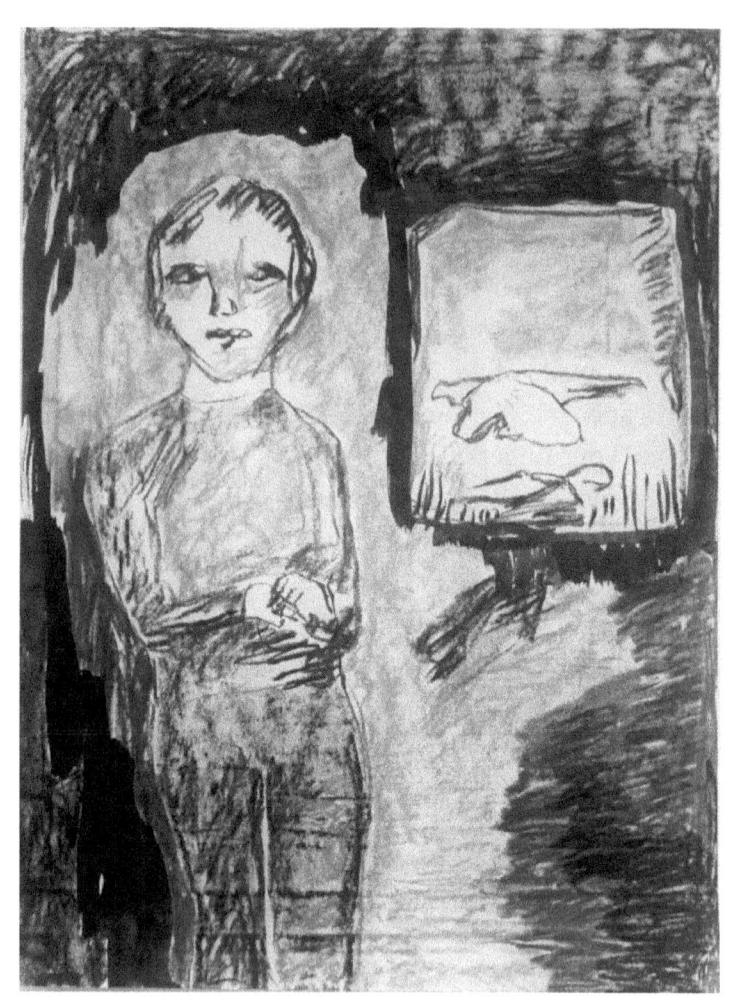

Waiting

A husband twists his ring
looks down from the window where
a dragonfly, transparent flutter
on a blue-tinged stick
hovers above a broken cricket
dragging through a thatch of grass.

When it rises up
sudden as a mind changing
the man's shoulders sag under
the last thing he wanted to see—
a pair of wings escaping
the world left out of reach.

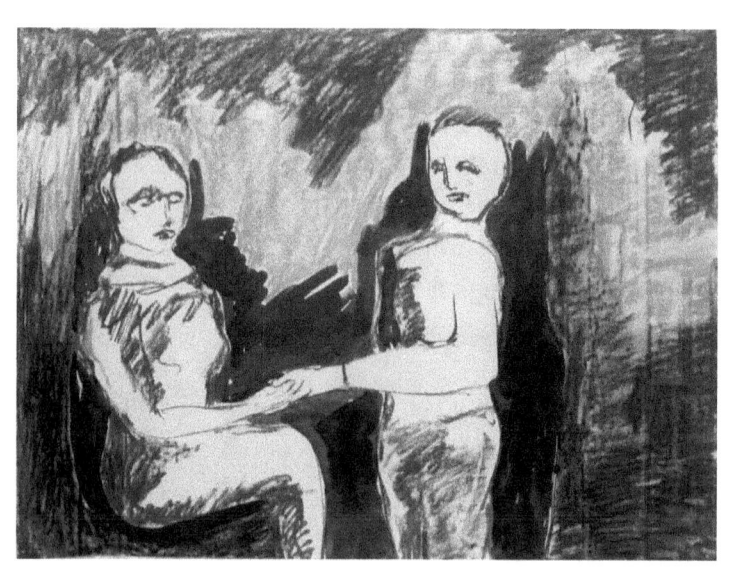

Recovery Room

She shivers awake
to find him
holding her glass fingers.
I'm still here, she whispers.
Her surprise cracks
over words too small for him
to pick up. *Where else would I be?*
he misunderstands
as if he hadn't run for miles
with her pulse in his ears. As if
she hadn't already said *goodbye.*

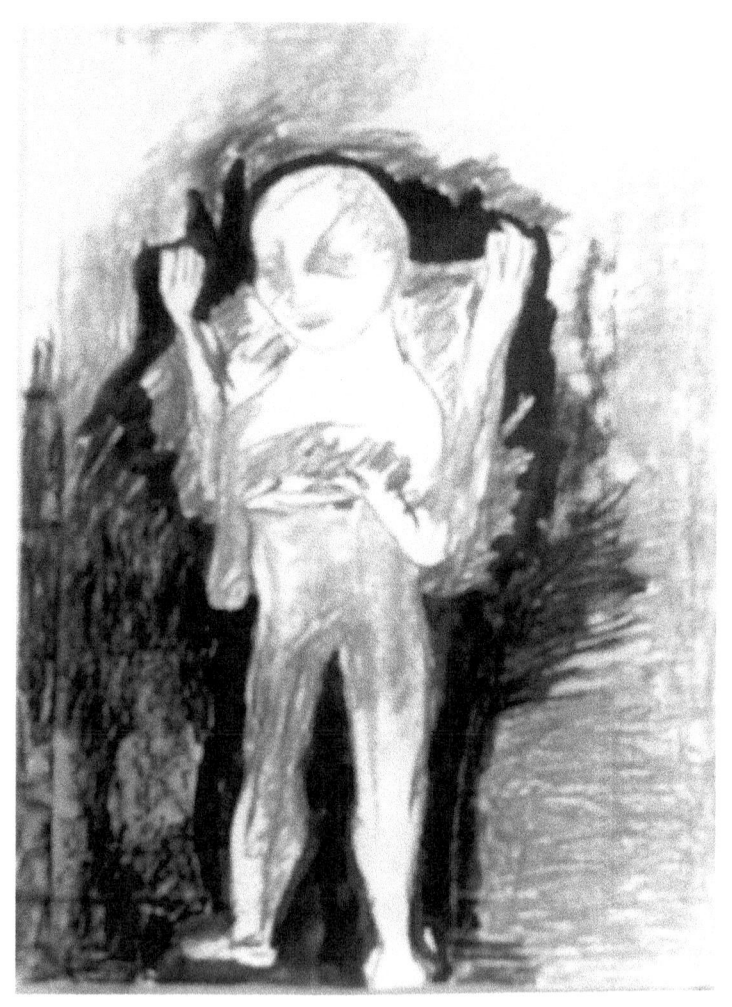

Scar

Every day you counted on his kiss to keep you safe.
Where do these ideas come from?

Think of his tongue, its long rogue lapping.
Imagine your newly-latticed skin, scar stuttering
along a ridge steep enough to fall from.

Remember that
the next time you place your faith in magic.

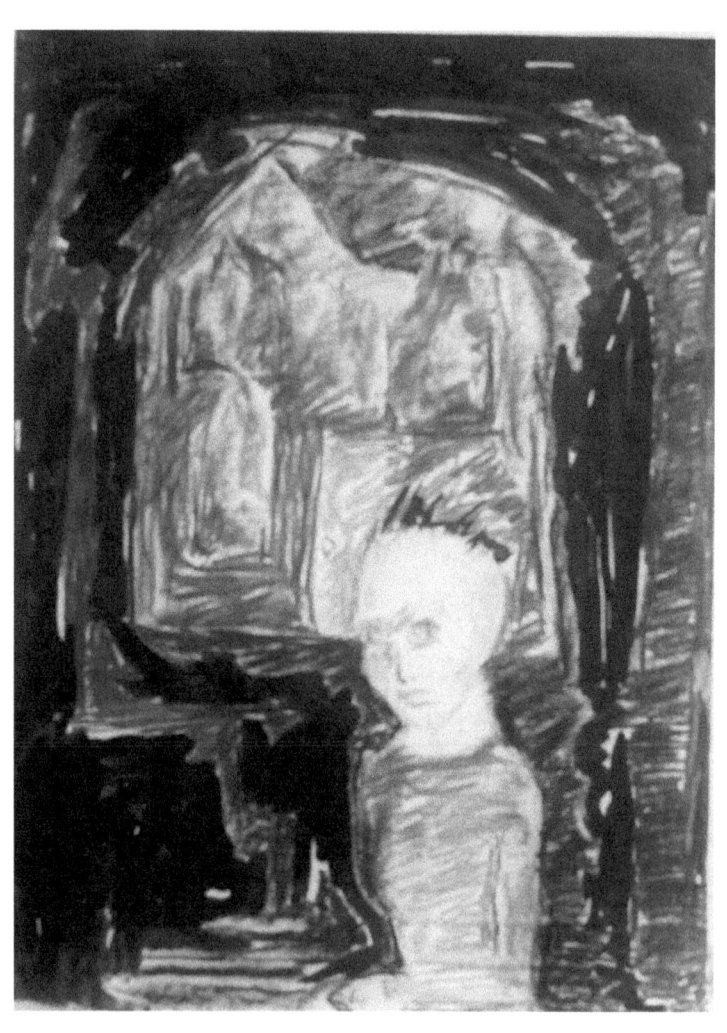

Radiation

Let's say what you want lives
with what you don't.

To put out one fire
you must set another.

A forest isn't needed for this.
A vaccine. The hair of the dog.

When it's kill to cure, a hot photon
spinning with contradiction

will burn through probability burning
through what holds you captive

in dreams of your house in flames.
and you climbing out free as a fugitive.

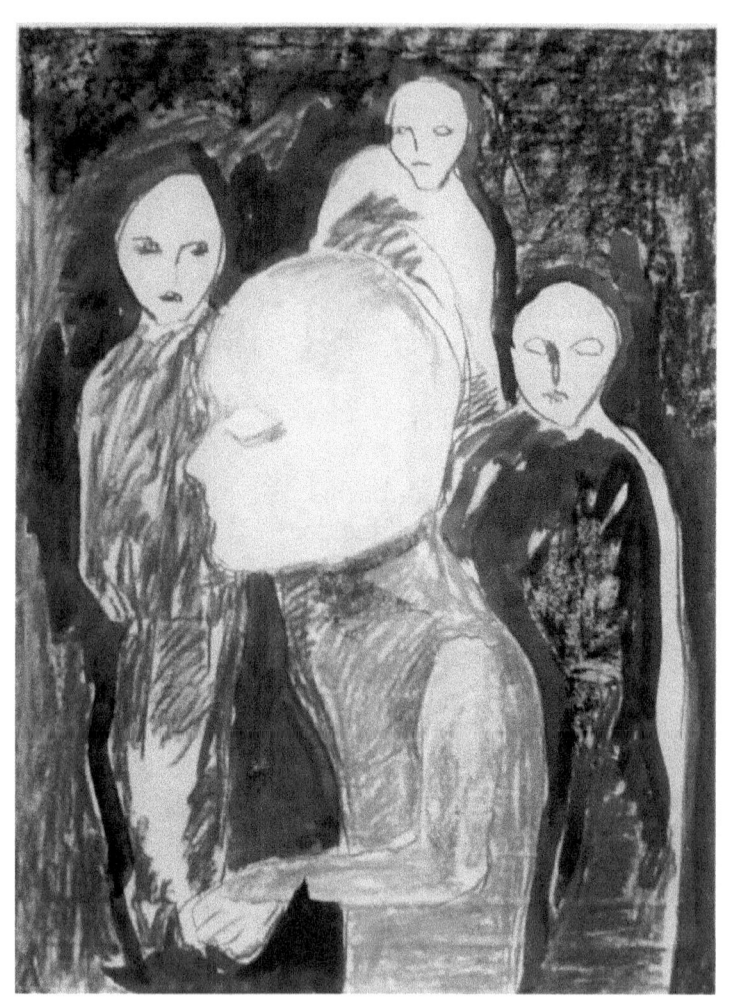

Aggressive

Don't talk to me about options.
When I say kill the cancer, I mean I want it dead.

Slash it, burn it, poison it without mercy
without stopping to sweep the hair from the floor

or scrub the red from the sheets. I don't care
about the tumor's grade and stage. Knock it down

to nothing the way people who see me coming do
turning from my limp and my lash-less gaze

blind to what it costs for me to stay here.

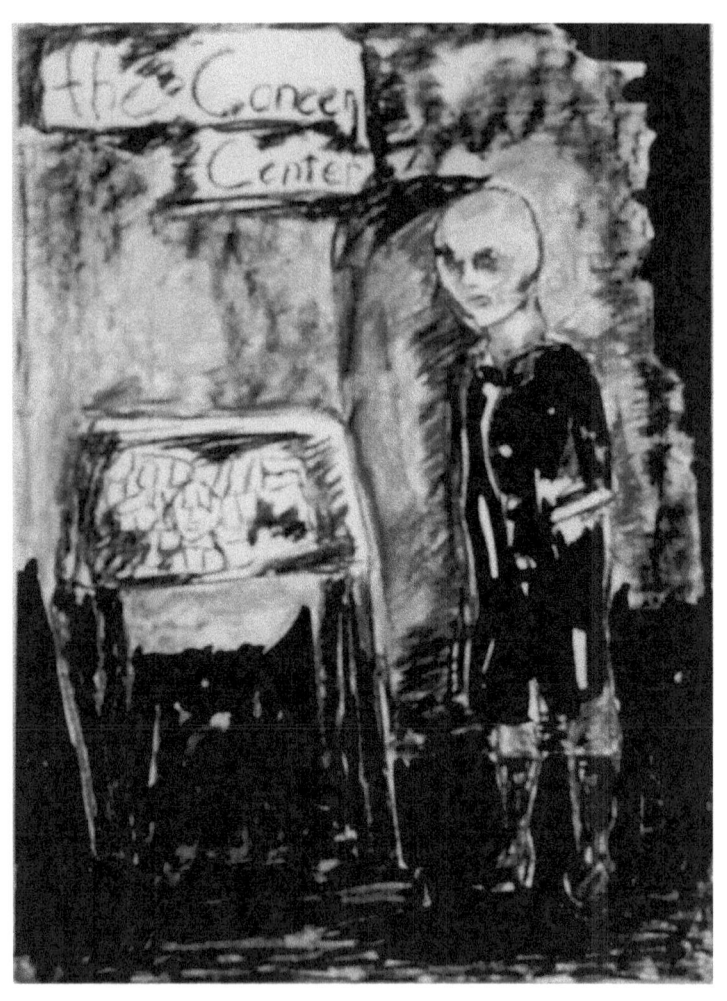

Blink

On the table
at the Cancer Center,
the jigsaw of a painting—
a staring nude
with two clothed men.
What are they talking about
as she sits in her vulnerable skin?
Neither will meet her gaze
so she turns her face blind—
until a patient steals her
and hides her in the winter coat
where she will no longer have to see
the brief space before death enters,
vanishing years filled with light.

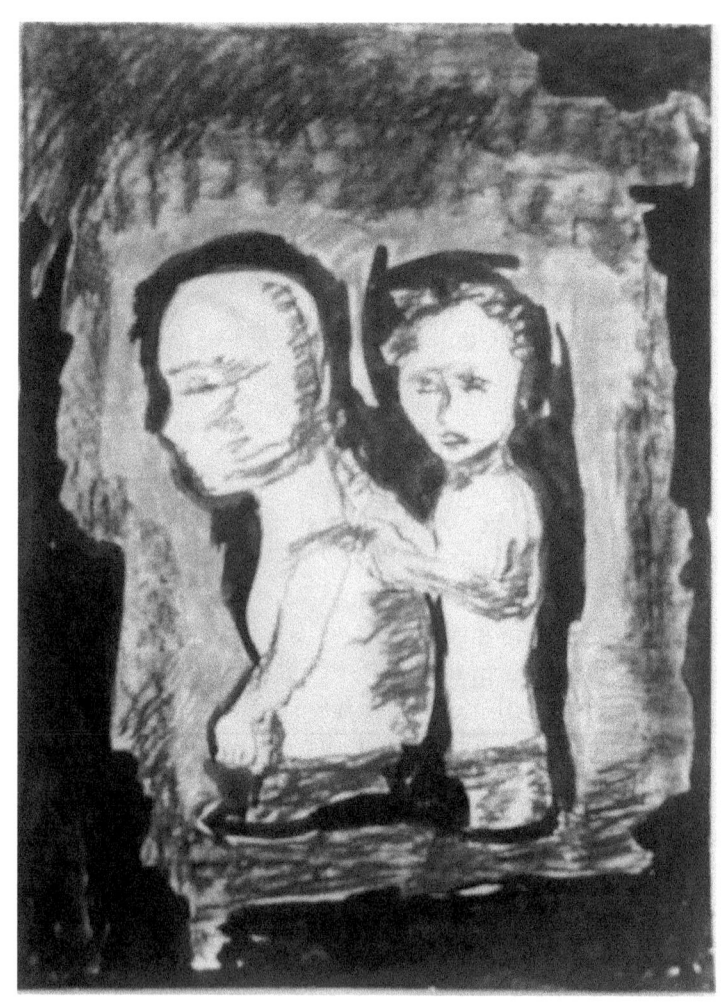

Circle Theory

You're better at last, your wounds
have closed, there is sapling strength.
Your friends think it's their turn now
though tit-for-tat was never established.
Demands are made. Some are met.
The ones who hurt you most
want forgiveness at all hours of the night.
You can't sleep through that, so when
one of them offers a backrub
when what you really wanted was sex,
you slide down your locked-out life
and count yourself among the lucky.

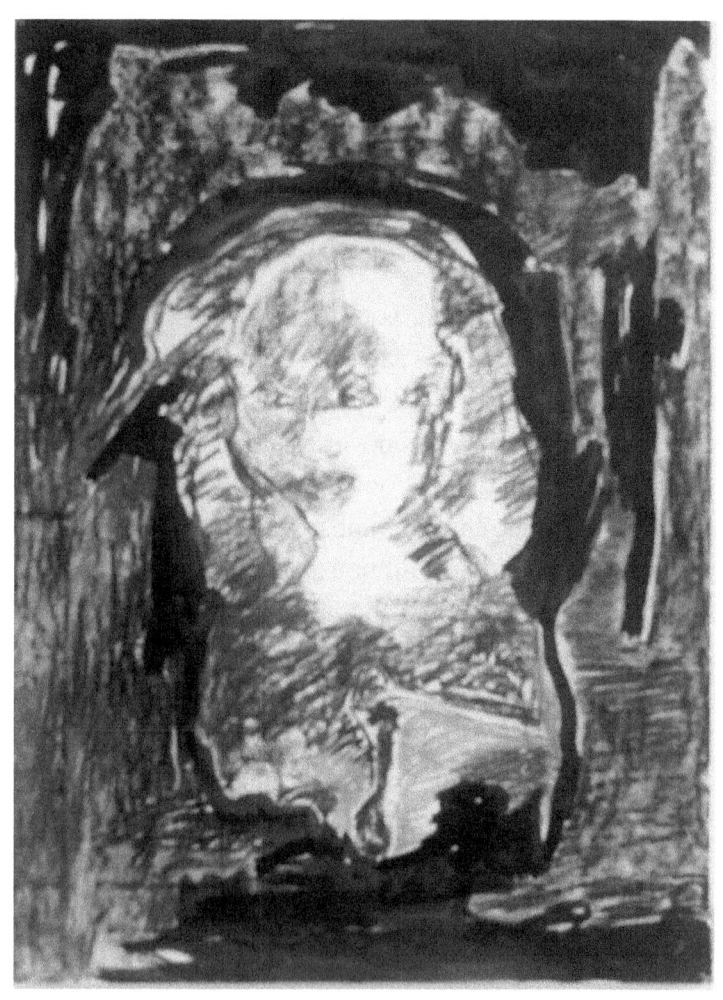

Afterimage

You should name it, this detonation.
The exploding star entered you,
sleeved its space around you,
molded its shape to yours
and now anything can fit in there—
beams from a mechanical sun
a catheter through the heart
poison dripping from a vial
the color of a bruise,
flooding veins that run the body
convinced it sensed a warning there
a warning it would recognize
if it ever feft it again.

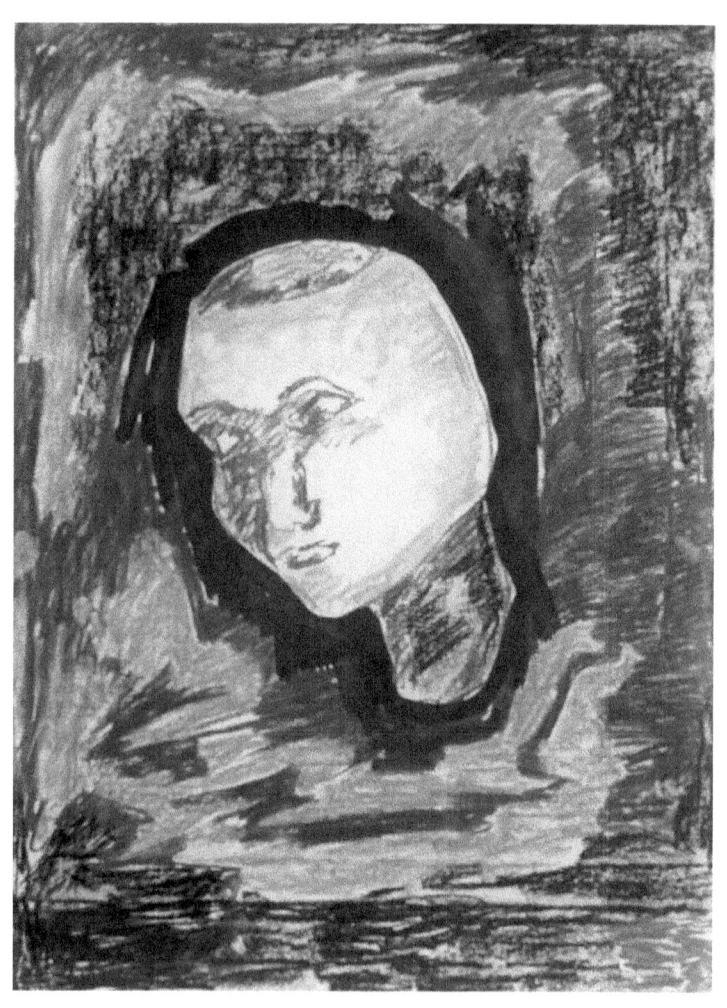

Reading the Hysterectomy Scan

disease may
remit

remission is
absence

absence is
curative

cure is
probabilistic

probability is
only a theory

in the face of
such widespread desolation

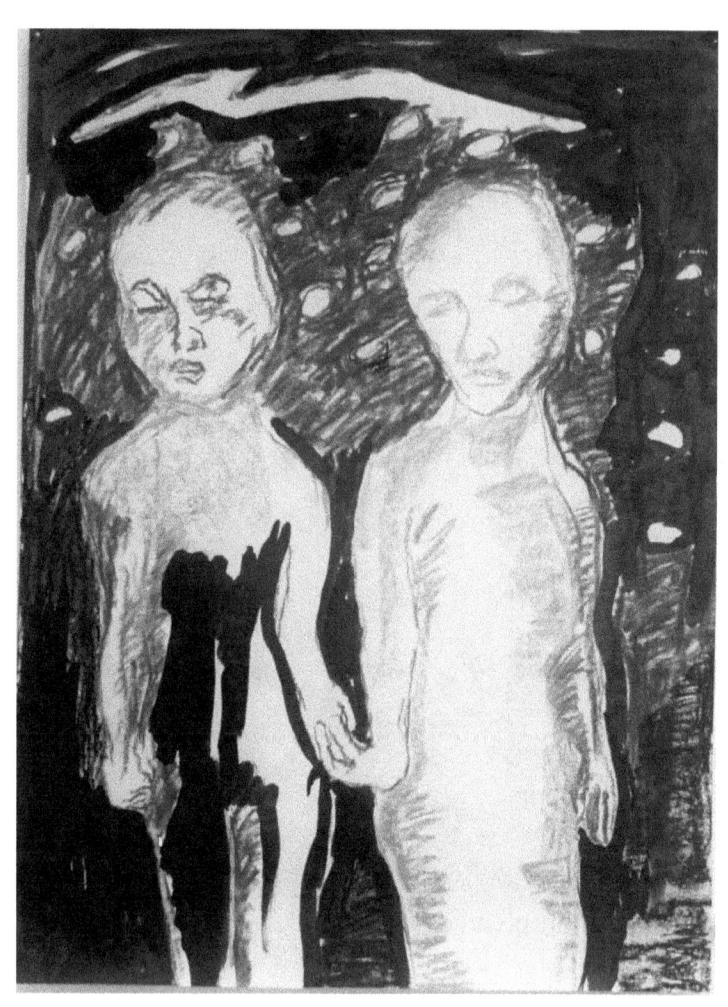

Recurrence

It's not like you'd think,
all abyss and crying. Last night
we held hands for hours—it's possible
to tune out thunder if the lightning is legible.
Under a ceiling strapped down with stars
you told me about luck—how it can
brush the edges of fate with change. I don't believe
in all that. We are made of death and dying—
stardust squeezed from the cosmos' vacuum
which is not so empty after all. Fluctuations
teem with possibilities—but I want you
to stop talking now. Let something come
from nothing. Let me tell you the truth
about absence.

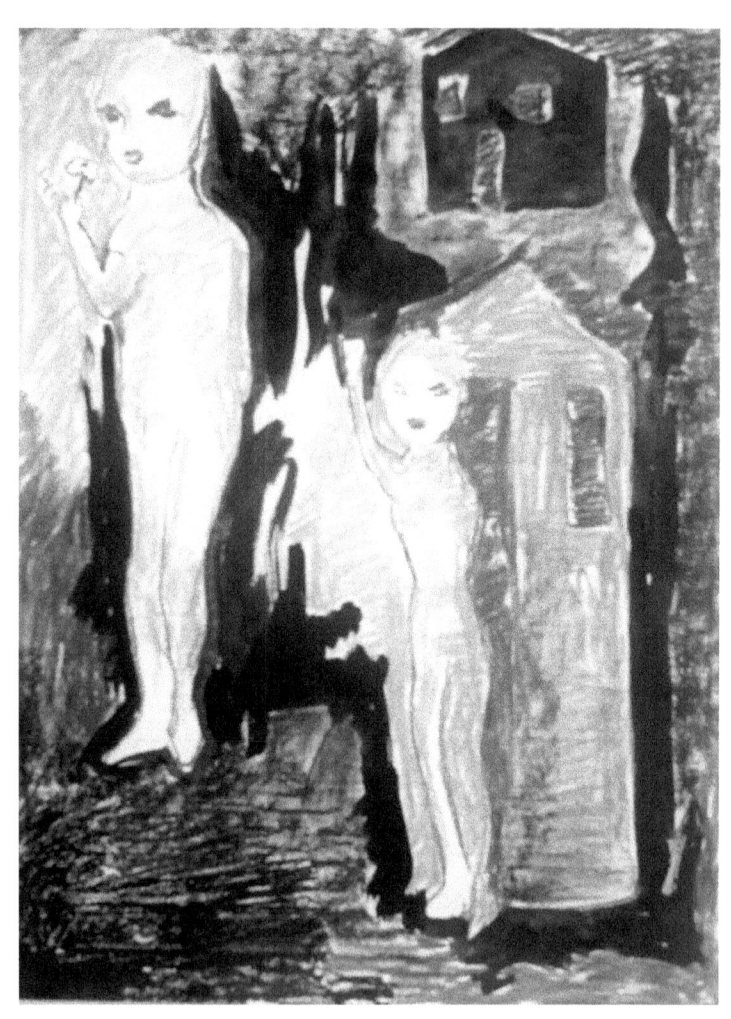

No Second Acts

The white bungalow. Falling-down steps
chalked with the secret messages of stones.
Cones of pink cotton candy, changing neon
telling how many burgers sold. Bad boys
with ducktails driving pedal to the metal
red coals of spent smokes flicked into air
stinking of rubber. The Goodyear blimp
above tall grass dented with shapes of summer
snow angels. Birds swollen with wedding rice.
Landlords and ladies. Wall-to-wall shag carpet
avocado green everything, sliding glass doors
opening onto the corner bar, afternoon motels.
A contract full of loopholes. Your diagnosis
the exit, once you realize there is nothing left
but the waiting.

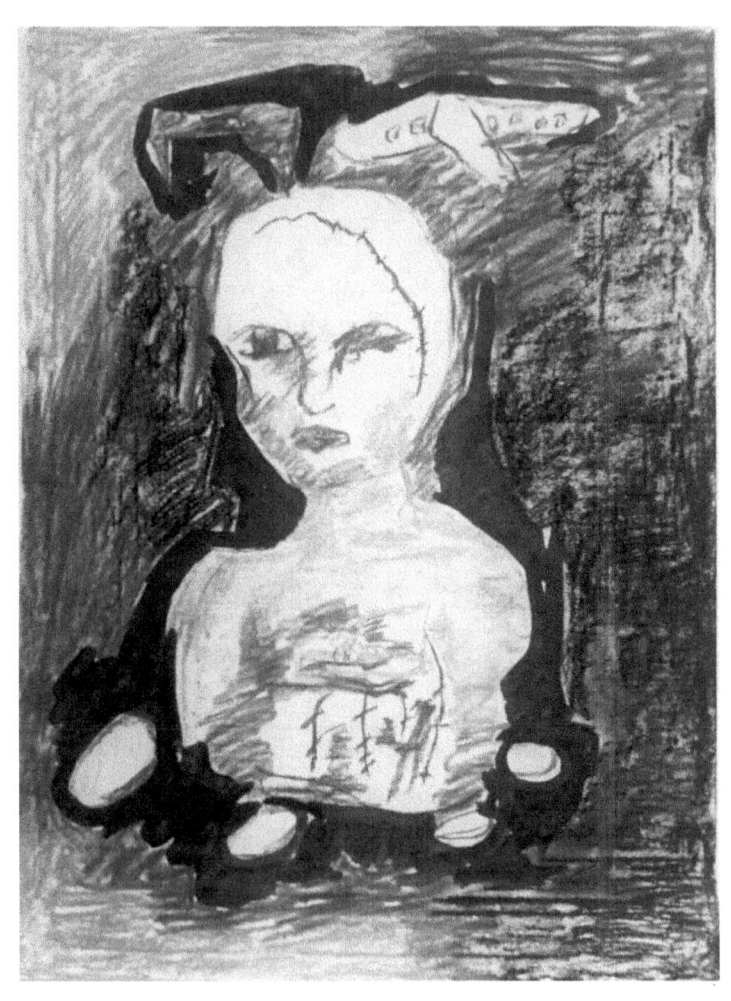

Unravel

Pull the thread and all the places
you wanted to see but won't now
show you other destinies
that might have chosen you.
A piano or plane falls out of the sky.
One train crashes another. Water
has always meant drowning
to someone but you could cash out
and go to Delhi or Rome, bills floating
from your purse into the foreign territory
outside Holiday Inn. You could pull
the thread through and open
your suitcase in some restroom
where to swallow stockpiled pills
would be to feel the final tug
of your own frayed will, the one thing
that could let you go still beneath your skin,
sirens wailing, blue and red lights spinning,
begging you to stop.

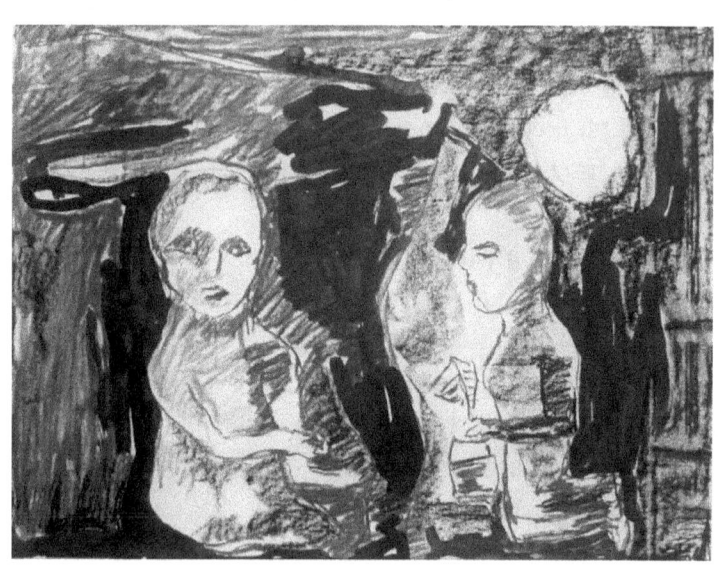

Alternate Therapies

She catches him kneeling on the shore
fishing with his hands.
I'll show you a better way, she says.

She opens a tackle box and he braces
for the worst, sucks air in behind
his teeth, rolling his eyes upward

to the sky where clouds sling
the sinking sun. She hooks a slick line.
Her lure is a thing with feathers and

he laughs at it, the sound scattering
the light. Later, when the sun bounces up
a moon, it's much brighter than they'd hoped.

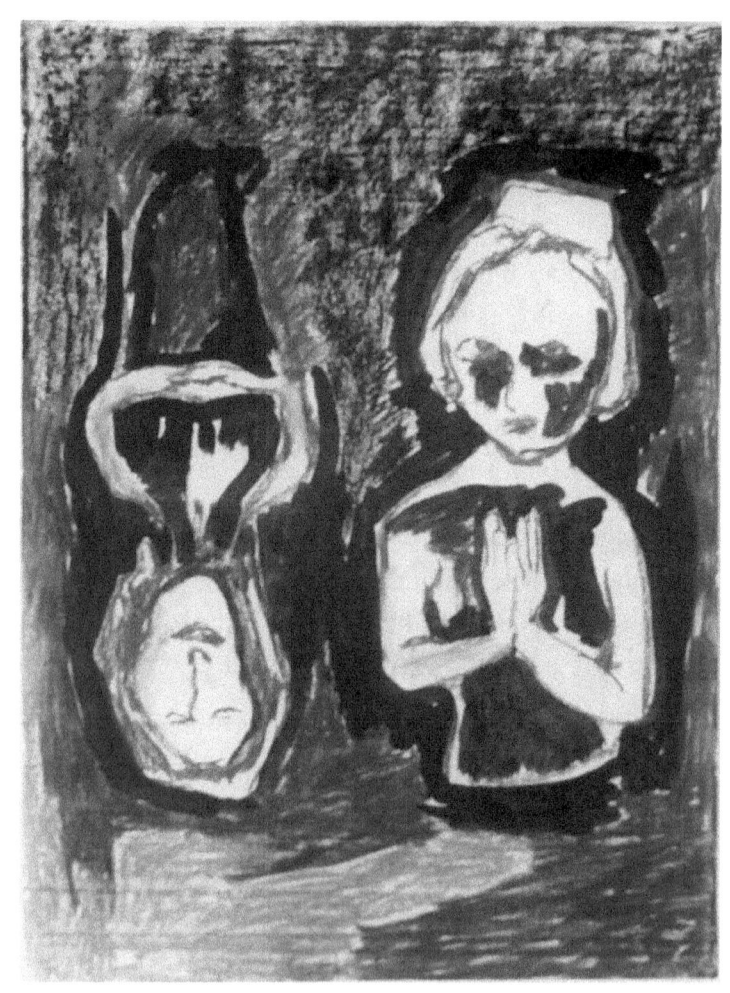

Faith

The nurse came in, thinking
I was asleep, and started to pray.

I wanted to throttle her words,
rob them of their power, but it was late
and I was weak from opening and closing
on a steel slab all day.

The next time I heard that prayer—
its cadence a flat-line static, its breath
the false thunder of rattled tin—
it sounded like a poem.

Faith sometimes comes across that way—
sliding in beside you with a blue mask on
wild with both sound and sense,
and you have to let it have its say.

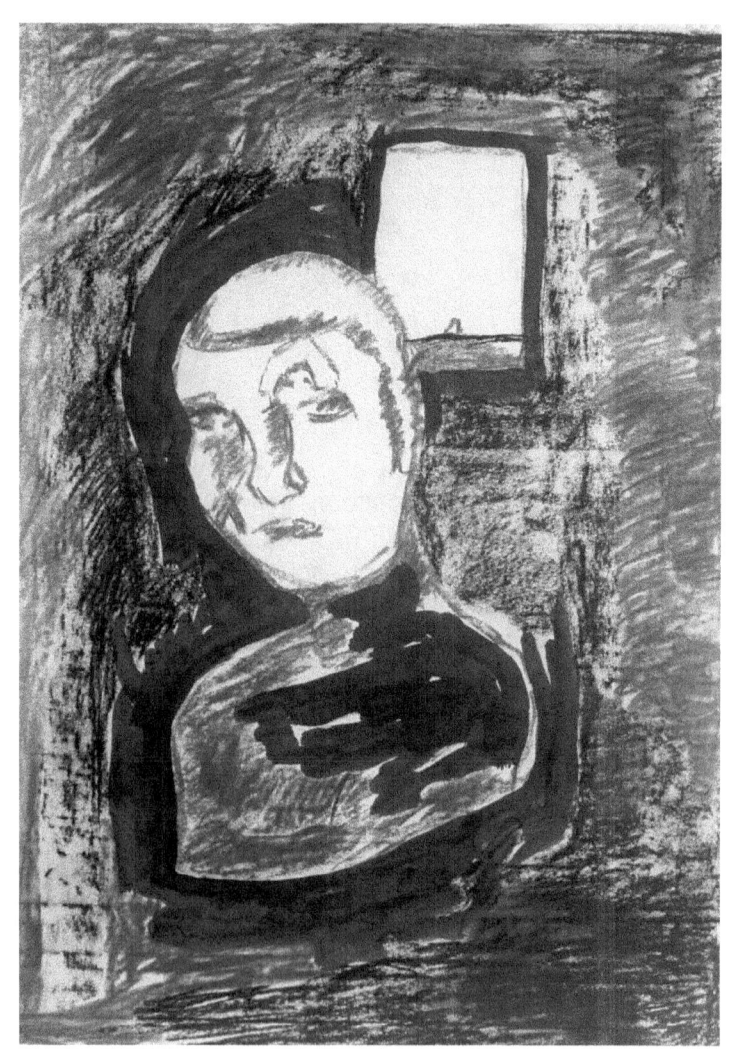

Survivorship

She thought she was a fortress
but cancer pitched a tent in her.

She cracked a window to let it out
but more cancer climbed in.

She tried to float above it
but the cancers poisoned her waters.

She rolled away like a fallow hill
but they had already seeded her.

She screamed at her body
as the cancers cut her out of it.

There was only one place
the disease had not invaded—

so the woman trudged up its steps
and set fire to every candle

 bearing her name.

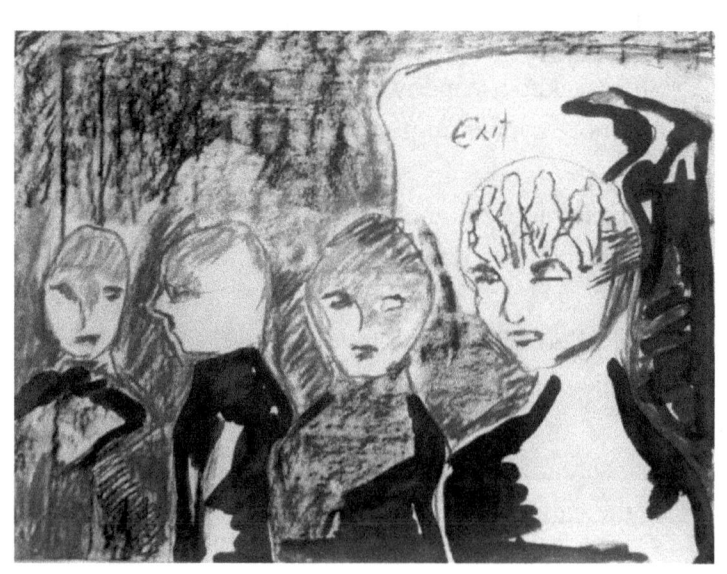

Support Group

In the room, she eyes the exit.
Next week she won't come
next week they'll miss her.
Well. Some will. Some don't –
outside the context of the room
she doesn't know who her friends are
and so searches aimlessly,
sometimes for months, until she forgets
what she was looking for. She'd like to
return to the room to start over
but others just like it have sprung up.
She enters the idea of the room instead
where strangers fill the seats inside her head.

They must have expected something fresh
after the big build-up. How were they to know
she'd already come full circle, beginning again
at exactly the point at which she thought
she was finished?

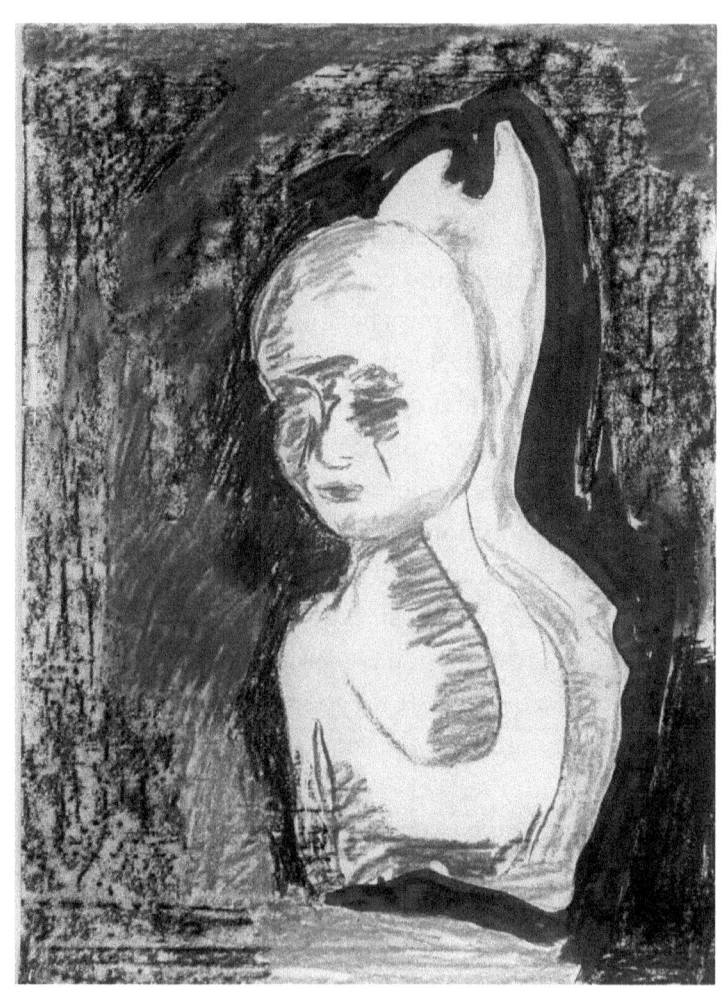

Late Effects

Light-fingered at first
by the time they are
everywhere they have
dug in
to loot the body
and douse what's left
with flames.
At night I wake
to ransack sounds
breaking bones
curdling blood.
I beg them to *stop* –
I can't lose any more—
but my voice is among
the lost things.

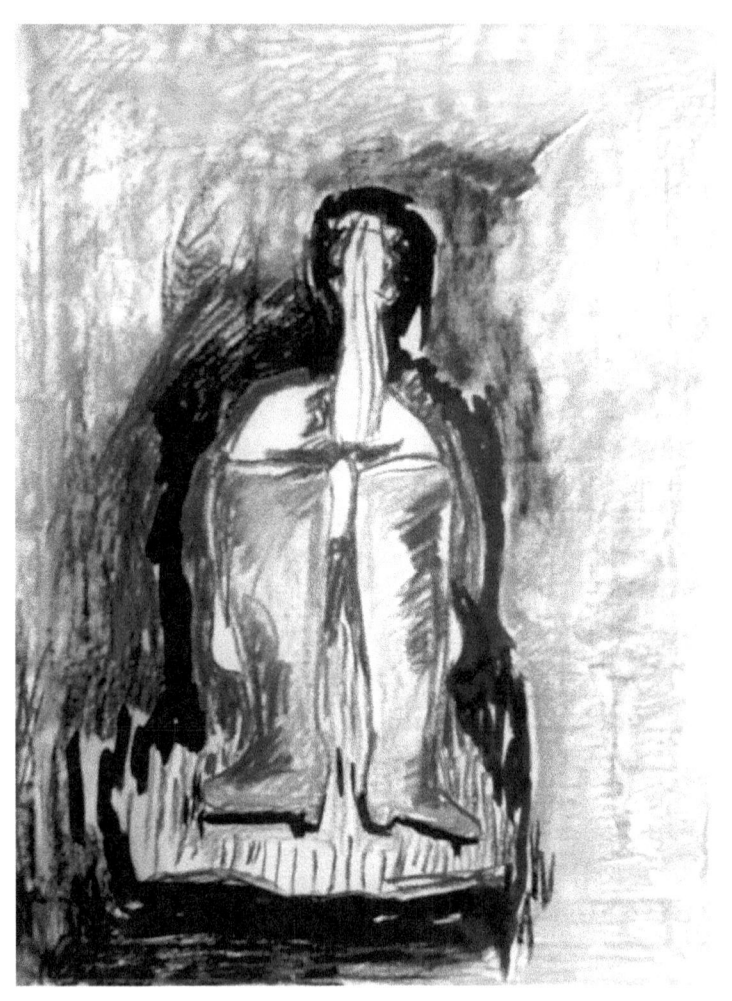

Anniversary of Our Narrow Escape

We go shopping for shoes
that may never be broken in
much less worn out. We can't dwell
on that. Too much reality
and our thoughts will go
to whimsy: a sudden desire
to learn the guitar or a dead language
hours spent poring over swatches
for curtains built to last. There's the conviction
that once committed to a big project
the time we need to complete it
will unroll like fresh turf under our feet.
Who knows how long that grass will grow?
There's always someone to tamp it down
with the old soft shoe
and the explanation that rescue
works best under a dark sky getting darker
the forecast filling with rain.

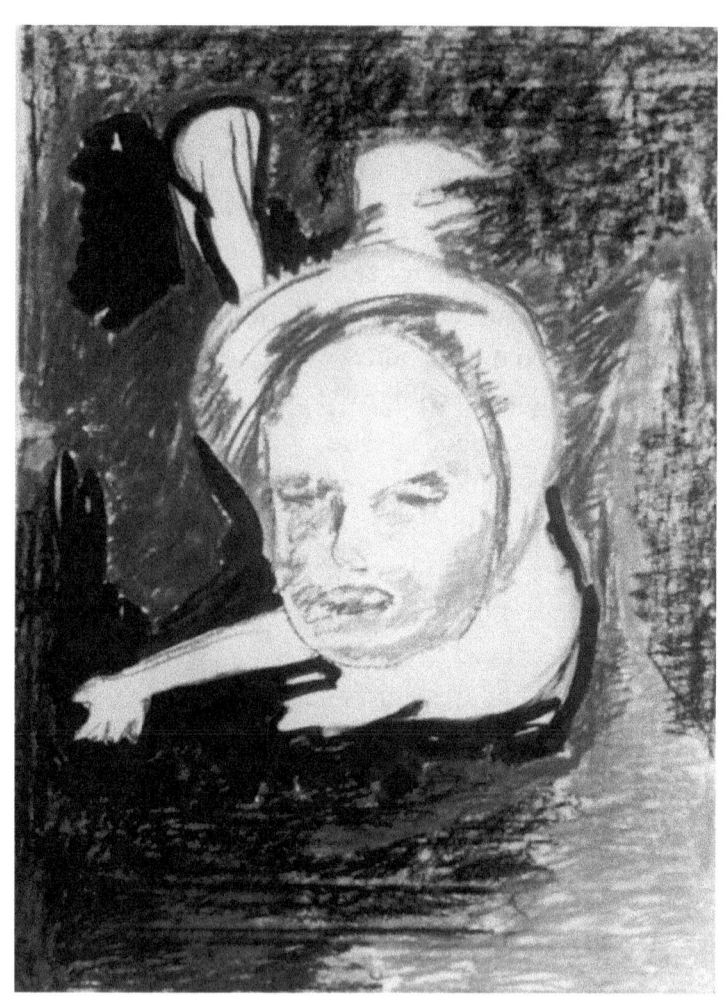

Where We Started From

The way somersault
circles us, so long stuck.
We stir the air with a doll's arm.

Oar, pull away. Breaker, tip us over.
Show the vantage point of the submerged
clouds wrong side up

Where we go who knows when
the knot gives way. Who, unlaced and dangling
can almost see the ground.

Other Titles by the Snell Sisters

Flytrap
Heads
Twice Told Tale
Shiva's Arms
Rescuing Ranu
Flower Half Blown
Epithalamion
Samsara
Multiverse
Prisoner's Dilemma
Variations on a Theme with Harmonica
Geometries